The Commonsense Guide to Abortion

Dispelling the Controversy and
Finding Common Ground

ISBN 979-8-218-58482-5

Dedication

This book is dedicated to sexually active teens and women of childbearing age who want to make the best choices for their bodies and for their lives, and to those who care about them.

Acknowledgement

Many thanks to Kim D. and Lynn P. for your valuable insight, time, feedback, and opinion.

CONTENTS

Why Common Sense?

Commonsense is something everyone has. It allows everyone to have something in common regardless of their diversity of opinions, thoughts, ideologies, or feelings about anything. We can agree to disagree on anything, but let us try to agree on the generic definition of commonsense:

Common sense - *sound practical judgement that is independent of any specialized knowledge, training, or the like, normal native intelligence. (Dictionary.com)*

Common sense - *sound and prudent judgment based on a simple perception of the situation or facts. (Merriam Webster dictionary)*

The old saying "Commonsense ain't so common," rings true today as in the past people are prone to allowing emotions, other's influences, and irrational thought overwhelm and overtake the value of interjecting commonsense into a given situation. Let us try to use a commonsense approach to the issue, the rights, and the facts of pregnancy and abortion. It will benefit women on both sides of the argument, which is what abortion should be all about anyway – the women that find themselves wanting to terminate their pregnancy.

This commonsense approach to abortion examines both sides of the argument, the facts, and the questions.

Word Usage Conventions

Because both sides of the abortion argument tend to use particular words or phrases for describing the same developing human being in the womb, a variety of choices from both sides were used. Pro-choice advocates tend to use words and phrases such as pregnancy material or pregnancy tissue, unborn, embryo or fetus while pro-life advocates may use the terms pregnancy, preborn and baby.

Big Question Big Proposition

Whether pro-choice or pro-life, isn't it possible that both could agree on the answer to this question:

"Is it better for sexually active women who do not want a child [at this time] to not get pregnant in the first place, rather than get pregnant only to abort?"

Think of a young woman not having to make the decision to abort or change her life by having a baby. Think about her ability to pay for an abortion or even find a provider, her mental health dealing with terminating her pregnancy, and the reaction of her family and male partner who contributed to the pregnancy. It is reasonable that most everyone pro-choice, pro-life, or apathetic would agree, yes avoiding an unwanted pregnancy altogether would be better than getting pregnant only to abort. Who would object to that if it meant that no one was trying to prevent a woman from having sex with whomever she wanted and whenever she wanted to? Though there may be many mothers and grandmothers who might advise their daughters or granddaughters against random, promiscuous, unprotected, or even unmarried sex it is still her body, her choice. There are so many choices to easily prevent pregnancy, why are hundreds of thousands of women choosing abortion over prevention?

Both pro-choice and pro-life advocates entrenched in their "rightness" sometimes result in arguments that lack simple commonsense. There are extreme views on both sides of the argument. Some pro-choice advocates feel a woman should be able to abort a human being at any stage of the pregnancy even up until birth while some pro-life advocates oppose abortion for any reason whatsoever.

A Proposition We Can All Embrace

This book proposes something else that both sides can choose to take a commonsense approach to advocate for reducing elective abortions by 50% every year through educating young women how and why to prevent unwanted pregnancies. As a society we could finally achieve what Bill Clinton embraced over 30 years ago (1992)- that abortion should be safe, legal, and rare.

Would there be opposition to this approach? Absolutely! Who would oppose women of child-bearing age to responsibly use contraceptives, know their body and ovulation cycle, understand what is happening during pregnancy, and what really takes place with abortion? Would mothers and fathers object? Would pro-choice or pro-life advocates object? Unlikely. The only ones who would be indescribably livid are abortion providers and anyone who profits from abortion services. Because as in many cases, money means more than lives. It is difficult finding data on how much money is made from abortions, but simple calculations result in conservatively over a half-billion-dollar industry based on medication abortions alone. In 2023, a year after Roe v. Wade was struck down by the Supreme Court, there were over one million abortions performed, which is on par for what it was previously. Most abortions are performed with medications costing on average $600. One can easily see how providers would not want to give up that kind of money if young women became more sexually responsible by protecting themselves from unwanted pregnancies. That knowledge would empower them to no longer be pawns of the abortion industry and those who vehemently argue for the right to abort anytime for any reason.

The Pro-choice Argument

Pro-choice advocates can be quite passionate about their right to end an unwanted pregnancy for any reason at all. Some may feel that the right should have little or nothing to do with what stage a pregnancy is at. They feel the growing baby in a woman's body *is* her body and she has the right to do whatever she wants with "it."

Pro-choice advocates arguments are generally:

- A woman has a right to her own body and the choices she makes for it (my body, my choice).
- A woman's reproductive rights should not be limited or governed by laws.
- Abortion is a personal reproductive choice between the woman and her healthcare professional, and maybe her sexual partner.
- Always allow abortion in the case of rape and incest.
- The government should stay out of a woman's choice for abortion.
- The embryo or fetus is not viable (able to live outside of the womb) until about 24-26 weeks.
- A woman often does not know she's pregnant for weeks or even a couple of months or more into the pregnancy.

- Banning abortion will result in women dying by choosing illegal abortions or having to travel long distances.

Their argument certainly has some merit since in the United States a woman does have the right over her own body. The fact that Roe v. Wade was a mainstay for decades and considered a Constitutional right, despite the opposition, aided advocates in enthusiastically embracing abortion. A female can use her vagina like a fast-food drive-through if she wants. Why should anyone be in her business about it? She can have as many abortions or babies as she wants. This too is her choice. The government and do-gooder Conservatives who oppose abortions need to back off.

Only if that life is growing and developing in the mother, which should be the safest place for the developing baby, do pro-choicers defend the right to cause their death.

And now for the other side of the story...

The Pro-life Argument

The reason pro-lifers care about abortion is that sexual intercourse produces human beings. There is no other natural way to create a person. Every one of us alive [and whoever lived] started out the same exact way – an egg in our mother fertilized by our father's sperm.

Pro-life advocates arguments are generally:

- The preborn are alive and human and no one has the right to destroy the innocent life except under extreme or rare circumstances (e.g., to save the mother's life, or fetal development with catastrophic abnormalities where it cannot live in or outside of the womb, some agree also in the case of reported rape or incest).
- What some call reproductive rights meaning the right to abort is actually reproductive death by definition.
- Women have numerous choices to avoid unwanted pregnancy and should be sexually responsible to prevent unwanted pregnancies rather than killing preborn people.
- Women do have the right to do whatever they want with their own body but once they [and a male] have created a life, does not that

12

innocent life who is *somebody,* also have a right to their life?

- The argument that women will die from abortion bans also speaks to their choices – a woman can choose to have an illegal abortion if she wants. She can also face the consequences of having created a human life without risking her life or destroying that of her preborn child. She could give away her baby at birth without even looking at him or her.

- Claiming a woman may not know she is pregnant until weeks or even months into the pregnancy, while true, is incredibly insulting to women as if they did not know they had sex and that doing it makes babies. Sexual intercourse is the **only** natural way to become pregnant.

Pro-lifers agree a woman has the right to do whatever she wants with her body. The sticking point is that after a pregnancy occurs, she is also making decisions for someone else's living, growing, developing human body. She is either a nurturing loving mother-to-be or an executioner of an innocent life. For pro-lifers, the issue is that once you have an embryo in your body that woman is growing a human life and everywhere else in our society it is illegal and immoral to kill an innocent human being for a "just because" reason or even a dog for that matter. Rational pro-life advocates agree that there are causes for abortion. If the pregnancy threatens the mother's life or when accidents of nature or other trauma causes the fetus to be medically futile, an abortion may be the most humane solution. Some can even agree with abortion in the case of reported rape or incest, especially in the case of minors.

Common Ground within the Controversy

There is a starting point which advocates on both sides so entrenched in their "rightness" could agree. It is likely that both pro-choice and pro-life advocates can agree that:

- Sexual intercourse between a male and female is the only natural way to create a human being and most young women of childbearing age know this.
- It would be in the best interest of a woman who does not want to have a baby at this time in her life to avoid pregnancy in the first place while remaining as sexually active as she chooses, rather than get pregnant only to abort.
- There are many effective methods to prevent pregnancy that are widely available.
- While a woman may not realize she is pregnant for several weeks, it is reasonable to assume she *knew* she had sex and if unprotected or her birth control failed, the morning after pill is legal in all fifty states as an emergency contraceptive without a prescription.

We might all (*except those who profit from abortion*) be able to agree that more education about ovulation, contraceptives, and fetal development could dramatically reduce the number of on demand abortions. We might all (*except those who profit from abortion*) agree that would be a good thing for women, and even for the men who did the deed but do not want the responsibility of a child.

More Questions

1. Why do you think neither side of the abortion argument emphasizes the fact that levonorgestrel, the morning after pill, (also known as Plan B and other generic names) is legal and available without a prescription in all fifty states and is 95% effective in preventing a pregnancy if used within 24 hours after sex? Would that not save a lot of grief, expense, and heartache rather than a young woman ignoring her sexual encounter until she finds out she is pregnant eight to twelve weeks or more after sex with a fully formed fetus alive and growing inside of her?

2. Since sexual intercourse is the **only** natural way to create human life. If you think about it, isn't a woman engaging in sexual intercourse without taking the precautions to

prevent pregnancy actually trying to get pregnant? *(Answer: Yes, she is)*

3. Why has there been no unbiased investigative reporting into why hundreds of thousands of women each year choose abortion over prevention methods that are widely available?

4. Why has there been no unbiased investigative reporting into who profits financially from abortion and how much?

Preventing pregnancy is not difficult. Planned Parenthood, the nation's largest abortion provider has over a dozen methods of birth control on its website along with their efficacy rates. Engaging in sexual intercourse without taking effective precautions and not wanting to get pregnant is like saying. *"I do not want to get wet!" and then jumping in a lake! Really?*

Our society must stop treating young women like idiots and expect them to use the intelligence and commonsense they possess to stop acting as if they are shocked and surprised they had sex then became pregnant! If a woman does not want to have a baby, she does not have to get pregnant, there are so many ways to prevent it. It takes education and a different mindset. It means understanding and respecting the incredible process of human development in the womb.

The Facts and the Choices

Given the over one million abortions (2023), why aren't more women choosing to protect themselves from unwanted pregnancies?

There are two major agencies who report abortion statistics, the CDC (Center for Disease Control) and the Guttmacher Institute. The wide differences come from how they gather the data. The CDC receives voluntarily reported numbers from state health agencies from most but not all states. The Guttmacher institute contacts every known abortion provider plus questionnaires from health departments.

The facts are:

- A woman's egg can only live up to 24 hours.
- Sperm can live inside a female up to five days.
- The only natural way a pregnancy can occur is for a female to have sex with a male who ejaculates sperm into her, and his sperm fertilizes her live egg.
- Once her egg is fertilized and before pregnancy occurs, all a person's genetic makeup is complete, including gender, skin color, hair texture and color, eye color, etc.

- With effective use of contraceptives and equipped with knowledge about her own ovulation a woman can easily and effectively avoid an unwanted pregnancy if she chooses to.

Are there really accidental pregnancies? A female must engage in sexual intercourse with a male at the right time in her ovulation cycle in order to become pregnant. She does not accidentally bump into a penis conveniently at the time she has a live egg ready for fertilization. It is a very purposeful act to create a human being!

So, why in our society are hundreds of thousands of women annually doing EXACTLY what it takes to make a baby successfully only to abort, get rid of "it?" Why does our society condone this behavior when there is a far better way?

Pregnancy is one of the easiest conditions to prevent. A male and female must do a specific act at the right time for her to become pregnant. Some education and contraceptives can go a long way in preventing every female who does not want a baby from making one when she *claims* she doesn't want one.

We now know how both sides *feel* and what they believe about abortion and the areas they could agree on. But we can hardly have a commonsense rational path forward without looking at the reason for elective abortions (a pregnancy) and how abortion works (how, when, where). We all must put on our big girl panties and look at the entire landscape to honestly evaluate and decide if the facts should make a difference at all. We must ask of the media, pro-choice and pro-life advocates:

1. Why has our society not placed the emphasis on how easy it is to prevent pregnancy and the many methods of contraceptives, rather than promote how easy it is to terminate a pregnancy?
2. Why have we allowed abortion advocates to ignore the fact abortion is the same as feticide, a crime, – causing the death of an unborn human being, but justifying it if the mother calls for the death?
3. Why won't both sides of the argument agree that pregnancy prevention is far better for a woman than facing the choice of abortion and come together to educate women and promote prevention to reduce abortions due to unwanted pregnancies?

Is "It" Alive and Human?

The scientific community leans towards presenting issues of humanness, life, and viability as complex, which often it is. But when we apply commonsense, native intelligence, to the equation is it really that complex or are scientists applying personal views and opinions to the equation? Study the weekly development of a human being in the womb and how you were developing in your mother's womb every day until your birth and decide if you were alive and human. How does something or someone not alive develop a beating heart, fingers and toes, internal organs, joints that bend and a body that moves, facial expressions, etc.?

Some place justification for abortion on the unborn because they are not viable outside of the womb with or without medical intervention. So what? An arbitrary measurement of viability is a feeble attempt to justify destroying an innocent human life. It does not take a lot of brain power to understand that it makes sense that a fetus would not be viable until a certain stage of development!

The scientific fact is that a fetus is a human body developing *within* the mother's body and it is also half of what the father contributed. Early in the pregnancy he or she has his or her own heart, internal organs, brain, limbs – their own body. The fact remains that to abort means that a little body stops developing and dies, not the mother but the unique *somebody* she was carrying.

Pregnancy Summary

There would be no abortions or people for that matter if there were no pregnancies. Another thing both sides can agree on! This week-by-week summary of pregnancy describes what happened in your mother's body after she had sexual intercourse and your father's sperm fertilized her live egg. This natural process is the same for every human being since people have been on the earth. *Sources-MayoClinic.org and ClevelandClinic.org*:

- **Weeks 1-2 (about 2 weeks after last period):** Your mother's body releases hormones for her uterus to prepare for pregnancy. Her ovary releases an egg. Sperm can live for 5-7 days in the female body.
- **Week 3** – Your father's sperm joined your mother's egg in her fallopian tube and fertilization occurred! Their union with 23 chromosomes contributed by her including an X chromosome and 23 contributed by him, (including either an X or Y chromosome) completes your genetic makeup including your gender (XX or XY) and physical traits; scientists call this one cell entity a zygote.

- **Week 4** – Your mother's fertilized egg travels down her fallopian tube and implants into her uterine lining where the placenta began forming. The now bundle of rapidly developing cells is a blastocyte. The amniotic sac forms to provide cushioning as her pregnancy develops.
- **Week 5** – Your neural tube (brain, spinal cord, neural tissue) forms and a heart tube beats at about 110 times per minute by the end of the week.
- **Week 6** – Your neural tube (along the back) is closing, and your brain and spinal cord are forming; your internal organs start to form. The areas for your ears and eyes develop and buds that become arms appear. Blood cells begin to take shape for circulation to start. Your heartbeat is detectable with a vaginal ultrasound. You are now an embryo.
- **Week 7** – Your bones and genitals begin to form; your brain and face grow and an area for nostrils and eyes begin to take shape. Lower buds appear to become legs and arm buds look like paddles.
- **Week 8** – Your major organs and systems are developing; your eyes are visible but still closed; your ears, upper lip and nose are forming, along with the umbilical cord which sends oxygen and blood to you. Your hands and feet form looking web-like, and scientists now call you a fetus.

- **Week 9** – Your arms grow, elbows appear, toes and eyelids are visible. Your taste buds, teeth, and muscles are forming, and your body looks like a baby even though your head takes up 50% of the length of your tiny body.
- **Week 10** – Your head is more rounded; you can bend your elbows; your arms, hands, fingers, feet, and toes have formed. Finger and toenails beginning; eyelids and outside of ears form.
- **Week 11** – You can open and close your fists and mouth; your red blood cells are forming in your liver and bones hardening; your knees, elbows and ankles are working, and your skin is see-through. Your external genitals are forming into a penis or clitoris and labia majora. You are about two inches and weigh about 1/3 ounce.
- **Week 12** – Your fingernails are forming, face is more developed, your intestines are in your abdominal cavity; your organs, limbs, bones, and muscles continue to develop. Your circulatory, digestive, and urinary systems now work.
- **Week 13** – You can pee and swallow; your skull and long bones harden; your vocal cords form. Your skin is still thin and translucent.
- **Week 14** – Your skin thickens; hair is beginning, neck is more defined. You can bring fingers to your mouth and turn your head; your external genitals have developed, and fingerprints begin

to form. You are about 3-1/2 inches and weigh 1-1/2 ounces.

- **Week 15** – Your intestines and ears move to where they belong, bones continue to grow, and your scalp and hair are forming; your lungs are developing; you are moving more and have facial expressions.
- **Week 16** – Your lips and ears developed, and you may hear your mother's voice; your closed eyes can react to light. Your skin is thicker; ultrasound can detect your movements. You are about 4-1/2 inches and four ounces.
- **Week 17** – You are gaining fat, are more active by rolling and flipping; your heart pumps about one hundred pints of blood per day. *At this stage, the mother can feel a flutter and it is often when she has her first ultrasound.*
- **Week 18** – Your digestive system is working; ears stand out and you can hear sounds, you have a sleep/wake cycle and may awaken to loud noises; your eyes begin to face forward.
- **Week 19** – You're covered with a greasy coating to protect your skin from exposure to amniotic fluid; your fingerprints are developing, and you can hiccup. If a girl your uterus and vaginal canal are forming, your mother can feel your punches and kicks.

- **Week 20** – You are regularly sleeping and waking, your nails have grown, and your brain is developing all five senses. You might be up to ten inches and weigh about eleven ounces.
- **Week 21** – Your limbs move frequently; your bone marrow helps produce blood cells; your sucking reflex is developing.
- **Week 22-** More fat is forming; your eyebrows and hair are visible; you can touch your ears and your grasp is stronger. For boys, their testicles begin to descend.
- **Week 23** – You are rapidly gaining fat, have rapid eye movements, your fingerprint and footprint ridges forming.
- **Week 24-** Your lungs have developed; your wrinkled skin is still translucent. You are about twelve or more inches and weigh up to two pounds. A baby born at twenty-four weeks may have a chance of survival with intensive care. *Over half of the states allow an abortion for any reason up to viability.*
- **Week 25** – You respond to familiar sounds (mother's voice) with movement; your body fat begins to smooth your skin; your nervous system is maturing.
- **Week 26** – Your body is making melanin determining your skin and eye color; your lungs

produce a substance (surfactant) that helps you breathe after birth.

- **Week 27** – You are gaining more fat/weight, can blink, and have eyelashes.
- **Week 28** – Your head may begin turning in the uterus. Your central nervous system controls your breathing and body temperature. You are up to fifteen inches and are two to three pounds.
- **Week 29** – You are kicking and stretching cramped inside your mother who feels your movements as poking.
- **Week 30** – Your brain is maturing, and you may have a full head of hair; your eyes fully open; red blood cells form in your bone marrow. You weigh up to three pounds.
- **Week 31** – Most of your major development is complete; you have distinct sleep/wake patterns and are still gaining weight.
- **Week 32** – Your toenails are visible; your skin is no longer translucent; you are getting ready for birth and weigh up to five pounds.
- **Week 33** – Your pupils can change in size responding to light; your bones are hardening, but your skull remains soft (to come through birth canal).
- **Weeks 34 to 37** – Your skin gets thicker and smoother, limbs get chubby, brain continues growing; you take up most of the amniotic sac;

your head starts descending down into your mother's pelvis.

- **Weeks 38 to 40-** Your head and abdomen circumference are equal; you gain a half pound a week and are full term. You are about 18-20 inches and weigh seven to nine pounds. You were born either early, on time, or a little late!

Six states allow abortions with no restrictions during the entire pregnancy.

Fetal Development by the Month

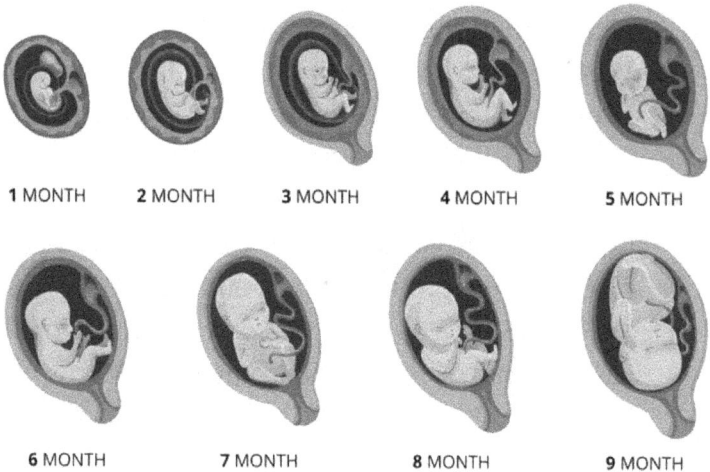

1 MONTH   2 MONTH   3 MONTH   4 MONTH   5 MONTH

6 MONTH   7 MONTH   8 MONTH   9 MONTH

iStock images

30

Is it not truly a scientific wonder how humans develop in the womb after just 39 weeks given the complexity of the human body and all its systems working in concert with each other?

Abortion Summary

Abortion laws vary by state, and some are in a state of flux at this writing, changing regularly with new legislation, lawsuits, and judicial decisions. At this writing nine states and the District of Columbia have no gestational limit on abortion. Twelve states have a total ban with some exceptions, which may allow for abortions to save the mother's life/health and or for lethal fetal anomalies. Seven states allow abortion from six weeks to 18 weeks. Twenty-two states allow abortion after eighteen to twenty-four weeks.

There are two types of abortion; medication induced (abortion pills) or in a healthcare clinic or facility administered by a healthcare practitioner, often a physician.

Medically Induced Abortions

The FDA approved medication abortions in 2001 as an option for terminating a pregnancy up to about - 11 weeks. Medication abortions take place outside of a medical facility, usually at home. Over half of all abortions now use pills to induce the abortion. It involves taking two medications. The first drug mifepristone blocks progesterone, a hormone necessary for the fetus to continue developing. The second one, misoprostol taken 24-48 hours after mifepristone causes the uterus to cramp and bleed, emptying the fetus out of the uterus and expelling it through the vagina.

This is what usually happens after taking misoprostol to hopefully complete the abortion:

- Bleeding and cramping begin within 1-4 hours.
- Heavy bleeding and cramping may take place for several hours.
- Low fever or chills for up to a day
- Other side effects may be nausea, vomiting, diarrhea, dizziness, or fatigue.
- Bleeding lessens and subsides over several days.

A follow up appointment with a healthcare provider within 7-14 days confirms the abortion was successful, usually by an ultrasound and/or blood work. Medically induced abortions are more successful earlier in the pregnancy. Planned Parenthood claims most pass the *pregnancy material* within 4-5 hours.

At the maximum ten-eleven weeks allowed for medical abortions that "so-called" pregnancy material has arms which bend at the elbows, legs, hands, feet, a rounded head, and that heart that started beating around 6 weeks.

In Clinic or Surgical Abortions

For abortions after 10-11 weeks, a surgical abortion must take place in a clinic or other medical facility. There are two types of surgical abortions depending on the stage of the pregnancy. Only qualified healthcare professionals can perform them.

Suction abortion – 12 to 16 weeks

Also called vacuum aspiration, this abortion uses suction to remove the fetus from the womb, which is discarded as medical waste or if allowed donated to a research facility. *By this stage, the baby has a working circulatory and digestive system, developed genitals, can suck their thumb, bend arms and elbows, have facial expressions, can react to light, and hear their mother's voice at about 16 weeks.*

Dilation and Evacuation (D&E) – Over 16 weeks

Practitioners use medical instruments and vacuum suction to remove the fetus (baby) from the womb. In states where late term abortions are legal the practitioner may first kill the baby in the womb before the D&E procedure. To quote the Abstract on *Induction of fetal demise before abortion,* by the National Institute of Health, "Inducing demise before induction terminations at near viable gestational ages to avoid signs of life at delivery is practiced widely."

After 16 weeks the mother can feel her baby moving around; the baby may have a sleep/wake cycle, can hiccup, and has his/her own fingerprints. They are continuing to grow, develop, and gain fat. By 23-24 or more weeks a premature baby might survive with intensive care.

What Happens After a Fetus Is Aborted?

Different states have laws, some confusing, regarding what to do with an unborn baby. With medication abortions done most often at home, the mother decides what to do. She may flush her embryo or fetus with the blood, the clots, and the rest of the uterine tissue (placenta, amniotic sac, etc.), or maybe she just throws it in the trash. With in-clinic or hospital abortion some states prohibit, and some allow donation of the fetus to research facilities but under federal law they do not allow compensation, except for the cost of packaging and transportation of the remains. Others allow for the mother to provide burial or cremation, while most allow for their disposal as medical waste. States vary on their requirements to counsel the mother on disposal methods or if they offer to give the remains to her for private burial or disposal.

What about Rape and Incest?

There are good and decent, not to mention extremely grateful people alive and thriving today who are the product of rape and incest. It's true. The story of Jaycee Dugard, abducted in 1991 at age 11, held captive for 18 years was repeatedly raped. She had a child at 14 and another at 18 by her captor showing the amazing strength of this young woman. Once freed she continued to love and raise her children. Amanda Berry was kidnapped, raped, and held for ten years in Cleveland, Ohio. She too had a child by her captor. Both women as are the countless nameless women who had and kept their babies or gave them up for adoption are proof that women (not all) are capable of separating the innocent child from the disgusting vicious act of the male who raped and impregnated them. That said, should a law force a woman or a girl to give birth to the innocent life that resulted from a violent crime, or should she have the choice to abort?

This opens a myriad of related issues from protecting our children from assault be it inside or outside of the family to punishment of the perpetrators. Giving children and young people the confidence to tell, **tell**, and **tell** until someone helps them, and never ever being afraid or ashamed to report the crime immediately is where we as a society fail miserably. Too often even the "nicest" families wish to avoid shame or scandal and want the victim to hush and forget about it while protecting their assailant when it involves a family member, clergy, or someone close to the family. The life-changing psychological impact from the assault whether pregnancy occurs or not adds to the burdens we often place on the victims of guilt, shame, and silence. We must support victims of sexual violence assuring them there is no guilt or shame on their part, only that of the perpetrator, only him, regardless of who he is (family member, respected member of the community, someone in an authority position). Pregnancy for a child or pre-teen may also pose complications to her physical as well as mental health.

Our Choices

The facts of pregnancy and the facts of abortion are clear, and there are many choices we can make to stand our ground or open our minds to consider other possibilities. We can all ask of each other regardless of which side of the fence we pledge our allegiance to:

- Do we choose to be more compassionate towards women facing the choice of an on-demand abortion or adamantly condemn them as baby killers?
- Can we choose to acknowledge some common ground on those who care about the human life developing in the womb or do we write them off as "do-gooder" religious zealots who won't mind their own business?
- Can we choose to encourage pregnancy prevention first over abortion regardless of which side of the argument we lean towards?
- Would preventing unwanted pregnancies by using contraceptives responsibly negatively interfere with a woman's right to choose how she uses her body sexually or would it be beneficial?
- What if the US led the world in preventing unwanted pregnancies? What would be wrong with that?

- Why not advocate use of emergency contraceptives (Plan B aka morning after pill) when unprotected sex or birth control failure occurs?

Are We Ignoring Some Things?

Over sixty million legal abortions have taken place since Roe v. Wade was upheld by the Supreme Court in 1973, making it a cultural norm. It also explains the backlash when it was overturned in 2022. Because something has become the norm does it mean it is right, moral, or best for individuals or society? Domestic violence, child abuse, gun violence are all cultural norms in the US based on their frequency. How incredible would it be if those things were rare instead of common place? Would we be a completely different country for the better?

We must deal with the fact that abortion and feticide have the same definition -death of an unborn human being. Does the argument of, "My body, my choice," lose some of its steam if we acknowledge the fact that the developing fetus is also *somebody* (with no choices)?

Let's also keep in mind that the mother knew she had sex even before the pregnancy began. What is wrong with advocating and strongly encouraging preventing unwanted pregnancies rather than destroying *somebody*? Are we calling it "reproductive rights" when abortion is effectually reproductive death?

Is it culturally hypocritical to insist on the right to destroy human life in the womb on demand when we abhor and criminalize it when anyone else takes an innocent life in or out of the womb?

The Extremes -Are Either of Them Good for Women?

Some states have all but banned abortion, allowing it only in extreme circumstances where the fetus or mother's life is at risk. They often attach criminal consequences to doctors and mothers if violated. In cases like this, courts should never make this medical decision. Extremists on the side of defending unborn life in these cases are threatening lives by allowing a judge or an attorney to decide a mother's fate. The simple, reasonable, and humane solution is that only the mother's physician with perhaps a second medical opinion should decide that either the fetus has fatal abnormalities or the mother's life is at risk by continuing the pregnancy. A court should not even be involved as the medical records should suffice. No judge should decide whether a mother's life is of more or less value than her unborn child's. These extreme laws are as

41

dangerous as those states which allow a woman to abort for any reason up to the time of a baby's birth. Neither of these extreme views have respect for human life or for women.

The Adoption Option

Could a woman becoming pregnant after consensual sex consider adoption? Why? Because there are tens of thousands of women who would give anything to be carrying that little life inside them, but due to fertility issues are unable to. They would take that little "it" in a heartbeat and try to be the best mom a child could have. And what a life altering gift that little "mistake" could be to a childless woman or a couple desperate to be parents. The cost is that the pregnant woman would have to hold her head high during her pregnancy and not care what others said or thought and give the child she is carrying and the adoptive parents a life they may never have otherwise. It may be the strongest, most compassionate, and selfless thing she has ever done in her life. While it may be a painful thing to do, abortion itself can also be a life altering painful memory that will not go away. It may not be the easy fix that abortion providers (who profit from it) tout it as, when there is an emotional price to pay.

The fact is we have relegated females of childbearing age to be irresponsible, while calling their behavior, "reproductive choice." Young impressionable females facing unwanted pregnancies often afraid, sometimes alone, buy the argument. Women of childbearing age have the ability and the power to keep abortion safe and legal, but to make it rare. That power rests right between their legs! With the right birth control, a box of condoms, and the morning after emergency contraceptive pill in the nightstand in case of birth control failure they could change the world.

Those who profit from abortion do not want women of childbearing age to take preventive precautions to avoid unwanted pregnancies. It would destroy their bottom line ($$$$) and livelihood if women on both sides came together for the cause of preventing unwanted pregnancies before they occurred.

What a Commonsense Abortion Policy Looks Like

As a nation divided on abortion, the truth is that a woman does not have to get pregnant if she does not want to have a baby. Before she chooses to open her legs, she can also choose to protect herself from an unwanted pregnancy.

No one is telling a young woman not to be promiscuous if that's what she wants or not to have multiple sexual partners or to abstain, although there are some mothers and grandmothers who might advise all three! On the other side there is nothing wrong with changing risky behaviors or abstaining for a time or even until marriage or at least until she is in a mutually committed relationship. How she shares her body sexually is her choice. She also has the choice to make wise decisions that do not result in an unwanted pregnancy.

Given that pregnancy is the development of a person in the womb, abortion being the procedure that destroys that developing person ought to be rare and specifically necessary. The reasons they are commonplace is because so many women chose pregnancy only to abort. Pro-choice advocates

44

would argue that a woman did not get pregnant on purpose. That is a hard argument to make sense of when a woman chooses to have consensual sexual intercourse, the only natural way to create a baby, especially if she is not using a reliable effective method of birth control correctly or uses emergency contraception afterwards.

A commonsense approach to abortion includes:

- Emphasize pregnancy prevention and contraceptives.
- Emphasize using the morning after pill within 24 hours after unprotected sex to prevent pregnancy and making sure it remains easily available (currently available in grocery stores and pharmacies in all 50 states).
- Require educating teens and young adults (females and males) about ovulation, conception, and fetal development week-by-week. *The week-by-week development of human beings should be widely known by all young people from middle school through adulthood by teaching it in schools, advertising it at every college and university campus along with where to obtain contraceptives, including the morning after pill.*
- Allow abortions at any time to save the mother's life if in danger or if the fetus has

suffered irreparable damage, trauma, or fatal abnormalities where it could not survive in the womb or after birth.

- After counseling to explore the facts and the options available, allow the choice for abortion in cases of reported rape or incest. A female should not be forced against her will to continue or abort a pregnancy because of incest or rape.

- Limit on demand abortions to before a fetal heartbeat is present or no more than six weeks. Why? Because sexually active females should be aware that they had sex, could be pregnant within days, and could have chosen to take the morning after pill within a day or two after sex.

- Require abortion clinics to be truthful and transparent about the stage of development the fetus is in [by ultrasound] and offer referrals to non-abortion pregnancy clinics who can help if the woman decides to continue the pregnancy and keep her baby or pursue adoption.

- Prohibit abortion providers from de-sensitizing and de-humanizing the truth with terms like *pregnancy tissue* or *pregnancy material* when referring to an embryo or fetus in the womb.

46

- Public education targeting sexually active females to encourage them to:
    - See their healthcare provider to learn about their ovulation (*when pregnancy is most likely*) and the most effective contraceptives for them.
    - Use contraceptives correctly and consistently (there are over a dozen choices of birth control).
    - Always use condoms with contraceptives if having casual sex or if not in an exclusive (both partners) committed relationship which may also protect against sexually transmitted infections.
    - Keep a dose of the morning after pill on hand to take within 24 hours in the event they have engaged in unprotected sex or if contraception failed.
- Public service ads on social media, broadcast radio and TV, billboards, subways and buses, health clinics, etc., on the many ways to avoid pregnancy. According to Planned Parenthood, below are just some of the ways to protect oneself which every middle school aged student to grown woman should know:

- o Abstinence – 100% effective (free but takes significant self-control and one mistake changes everything)
- o Implant, IUD, vasectomy (male) or tubal ligation (female) – 99% effective
- o Birth control shot – 96% effective
- o Birth control patch, pill, or vaginal ring – 93% effective
- o Diaphragm or condoms – 87% effective
- o Spermicide and gel or birth control sponge -78% to 86% effective
- o Cervical cap 71 -86% effective
- o Withdrawal (78% effective) or Fertility Awareness (77-98% effective)
- If abortion providers receive taxpayer dollars also equally distribute it to pregnancy centers who do not provide abortions but support a pregnant woman throughout the pregnancy and into parenthood, provide contraceptives, counseling, pre-natal care, and adoption alternatives.

It is anti-woman and anti-life to promote abortion and not emphasize the many choices to prevent unwanted pregnancies.

Commonsense tells us that destroying a developing innocent human life should be taken more seriously than "I don't want it," "I made a mistake," or reasons other than involving the mother's life and health or if there are abnormalities where the baby's death is inevitable in or out of the womb. In other words, commonsense tells us abortions should be rare rather than commonplace. So, for whatever reasons a young woman chooses to use her body she can still be smart and make the choice to prevent an unwanted pregnancy.

Why aren't both warring sides (pro-choice, pro-life) coming together to say, "Let's make abortion rare by showing women the many ways to protect themselves from unwanted pregnancies?"

The message of prevention needs to be widespread in mainstream media, social media, in schools and colleges, on billboards! See a bus rolling down the street with an ultrasound image of a baby in the womb sucking its thumb or hear this on the radio or see it on TV-

It is super easy to avoid an unwanted pregnancy and avoid an abortion. Be responsible, talk to your healthcare provider today about your many contraceptive options to avoid an unwanted pregnancy! If you make a mistake, take the Plan B morning after pill which is most effective

49

within 24 hours after sex, and available at grocery stores and pharmacies.

There will always be a reckless young woman who is under the influence of something and has meaningless sex regretting it the next day while nursing her hangover. She would be the one not to be on contraceptives, failed to use a condom and doesn't know where she is in her ovulation cycle. She would be the one a few weeks later throwing up and realizing her period is late, scared to tell her parents or the father if she knows who he is, then seek an abortion. With a little forethought she too could avoid an unwanted pregnancy or at least have the morning after pill on her nightstand ready to swallow the day after her escapade.

Is Preventing Pregnancy Better Than an Abortion?

Sounds like a dumb question, doesn't it? When asked so plainly and unemotionally, commonsense obviously says yes, it is smarter, cheaper, less emotional, less stressful to prevent an unwanted pregnancy rather than getting pregnant and then destroying the life just created. Makes perfect sense, right? Why do hundreds of thousands of women annually get pregnant only to say they do not want a baby? The right-wing religious crowd would say that's why fornication is a sin! If young women weren't having unmarried sex all over the place, they wouldn't be killing their preborn babies and catching all kinds of sexually transmitted infections (STIs) too. There may be some truth to that whether we like it or not, but it certainly isn't going to stop unmarried women from having sex. So regardless of what one believes morally about sexual activities, how could we all help women who aren't ready to have a baby, prevent getting pregnant rather than facing a decision to abort, keep or give away the baby they created?

What is the excuse of young women in the United States, when even the corner gas station carries condoms, and pharmacies and supermarkets everywhere have at least a shelf if not an aisle with over-the-counter contraceptives? There are healthcare providers, community clinics, and physicians who can prescribe the various kinds of birth control. The information is on the internet with a simple Google search, and since women of childbearing age are not inherently or hopelessly stupid, why have over one million abortions taken place (2023)?

Our society has failed young women in their most vulnerable state, and instead given them a band aid to "fix" their unwanted pregnancy, at their emotional expense and to the profit of the abortion industry. A teen or young woman having a consensual sexual encounter may upon finding herself pregnant look back in hindsight and realize that "fun" encounter has changed her life, and it was not even that much fun, and certainly not worth the predicament she finds herself in. Does she feel her decision was *well worth it* now that she is facing either having a baby to keep or give away or as hundreds of thousands before her decide to destroy *who* she created? Or does she look back and see how easy it would have been to skip the "fun" that day until she could properly protect herself from pregnancy? Young women need to know that sex is not going anywhere ever! If you do not have sex today, this week or this month, it will still be around and it is usually quite easy to find someone who is more than willing to do it with, especially without a commitment.

Women can and should become smarter about their choices. A woman does not have to choose an abortion if she makes wise choices to insure she does not get pregnant in the first place. It is entirely reasonable and doable.

A sexually active woman of childbearing age has a choice [and a responsibility] to protect herself from use for someone else's pleasure at the expense of creating a new but unwanted life. The wonderful thing about the many prevention choices is that she will not have to decide to end a life.

What is wrong with both pro-choice and pro-life advocates coming together to promote pregnancy prevention with the various contraceptives available instead of vehemently screaming their views at each other?

Wouldn't that be in the best interest of women's health? While a man may tell his partner that it doesn't *feel* the same with a condom, a woman's intelligent response should be *"neither does an unwanted pregnancy,*" reminding him that he can't get pregnant, nor would he have to make the decision to end one. If young women would simply think ahead of time before having sex and ask themselves, *"If I get pregnant then wanted an abortion or contracted an incurable disease through sex, was the pleasure of the sexual encounter worth a pregnancy, an abortion or lifetime medication?"* Parents, teachers, clergy, should pose these questions to young women. While sex can be wonderfully pleasurable, what pleasure would be worth the negative consequences of pregnancy or disease when a little pre-planning could avoid both? Women must act as smart as we know they are, and stop being manipulated by those factions who profit from [abortions] and prey on their emotional and vulnerable state once they find themselves pregnant and not wanting a baby.

In July 2023, the FDA approved Opill®, the over-the-counter birth control pill that will be available without a prescription and without age restrictions as this writing. It is difficult to find good excuses for women engaging in consensual sex to not use one or more of the many preventative methods to avoid unwanted pregnancies.

Culture and Abortion

Social narratives are highly manipulative and often target the vulnerable. Too often they are not rooted in the whole truth or commonsense, but in the ulterior motives of those pushing their narrative. The cultural messages of abortion are that unborn babies do not matter, are not really alive or human, and "it" is just "pregnancy material or tissue" [with a heartbeat, a brain, arms, feet, and legs all by 9-12 weeks!]. So how did we get here? The *free love* movement in the 60's and 70's embraced non-committed sexual relationships often with multiple partners. Women adopted an attitude that if a guy can do it so can they. Birth control pills were on the market, and in 1973 the Supreme Court upheld Roe v. Wade. With women seeking more equality they also associated it with sexual freedom, or so-called sexual freedom while we ignored the consequences of sexually transmitted infections, some incurable, unwanted pregnancies and abortions, or children born into single female households, too often in poverty. Where is the freedom for women in all of that?

We forgot that with freedom comes responsibility and that females and males are different – physically and mentally. The uterus, found only in females is the only natural place for a person to develop and be born from. Sexual intercourse at the right time of the month for a woman is the only way to naturally make a baby. A female can have sex one time and become pregnant (even her first time), while a male can have sex every day for the rest of his life and never ever become pregnant. Duh!

Women can sometimes (not always) feel an emotional attachment sooner than men after having sex. The woman may think she is in a relationship when the man may think how easy she was to have sex with and delighted she isn't looking for a commitment. He's glad he didn't have to work for it or bother to get to know her since she was a willing booty call - no harm no foul. Our baby boomer relatives would claim she is *giving away the milk for free*! The males who enjoy uncommitted sex calls *her* a booty call.

Sexually active men may agree with the idea of women being freer with their bodies and having the option of abortion if they "made a mistake." Why wouldn't they? Had their grandfathers impregnated someone in their day both of their families might have forced the couple to marry to avoid the shame of having a child out of wedlock! There was also the illegal abortion option which women took, risking their own lives to avoid the shame of having a baby and not being married.

Culturally we have de-sensitized women of childbearing age to value the life inside *their* womb. We have made it "Ok" to perpetuate the hypocrisy of valuing that life if a woman is happily "expecting" a baby and to de-value that life and "get rid of it" if she does not want her baby. It is the same human baby developing in its mother, just a different attitude of the mother towards her own flesh and blood, which means life or death.

If abortion were not profitable to abortion providers, pregnancy prevention would be the name of the game. Money takes precedence over what is best for women. With hundreds of thousands of abortions performed annually there is a lot of money involved. Why would an abortion clinic, even those who provide other services promote and encourage prevention over abortion?

A woman is often scared and vulnerable when facing an unwanted pregnancy. At that point she may regret not having used proper protection, even regretting the sexual partner she chose, but she is pregnant now and does not want a baby. The fun and pleasure of the sexual encounter is suddenly not worth the result, and she knows that life would have been simply fine if she never did it at that time in the first place. Teens and young women often panic. They fear telling parents or the father [who was a full participant in the act]. They think of all the things they should have thought of prior to having sex and now they face the decision. It's easy to think how simple it would be to just get it over with, abort and go on with life.

All the while that little life is rapidly growing and developing, making time of the essence. Pregnancy centers that do not perform abortions can help a pregnant woman decide what her options are, offer support if she chooses to have and keep her baby or give it up for adoption. Pregnancy centers may provide post abortive counseling if a woman chose abortion, then has regrets or mental health issues afterwards. They provide support throughout and well beyond the pregnancy with baby supplies and assistance to help the mother become a good parent.

You never saw any advertising by abortion clinics or government agencies like the Department of Health and Human Services, or the Office of Women's Health that encouraged women to be sexually responsible enough not to create a human life that they do not want. Never have you heard a public service announcement or advertisement saying- *"Reduce abortions- Learn your ovulation, learn how pregnancy occurs and how a baby develops in the womb, choose the best contraceptives recommended by your healthcare provider. If you make the choices and take the actions to not get pregnant, you won't have to face choosing an abortion."*

What a difference education makes! The problem is the profitability of abortion. Sadly, the scared vulnerable women and their preborn babies pay the price, literally and figuratively.

National Review reported that Planned Parenthood performed over 383,000 abortions in 2021 about 8.5% more than the previous year making up over 40% of the abortions performed in the United States. At the same time, their other services like cancer screenings, well woman tests, sexually transmitted infections testing and even pregnancy testing fell dramatically. The organization boasting over six hundred centers in the US receives over a half billion of our tax dollars in funding and grants to assist with providing low-income women with health services. Yet they are the nation's largest abortion provider, when tax dollars instead could be allocated for them to be the nation's largest preventer of unwanted pregnancies!

Pro-abortion advocates argue that the Supreme Court decision that overturned Roe v. Wade threatens women's rights and health. Because women have the right to become pregnant, do they not also have the responsibility to not get pregnant (creating a human life), rather than claiming an "unwanted pregnancy"? A woman knows she had sex, and that pregnancy is a possibility. Why should she *not* take the proper precautions to prevent the pregnancy?

Women, Race and Abortion

The rate of abortion among Black women (38%) and Hispanic women (33%) is higher than that of White women (21%). The Guttmacher Institute, CDC, and National Institute of Health report essentially the same rates. Yet women regardless of race who seek an elective abortion do so because of an unwanted pregnancy. There are many reasons such as lack of access to contraceptives, education, healthcare options, poverty, etc. for why women of color have higher rates of unwanted pregnancies. Only the Black and Hispanic community can reduce these rates by increasing access to contraceptives, educating females to get pregnant only when they want to have a child and using preventative methods when they do not want one. Otherwise, these rates will remain the same as they have for years.

Is the Media Biased?

Sadly, the media often reports the abortion issue in a biased manner in mainstream media outlets. You will never see a mainstream media journalist ask:

- Doesn't a woman know when she has sex and that she could get pregnant?
- Couldn't the morning after pill have prevented hundreds of thousands of those abortions? Why do you think it wasn't used more?
- Why would any woman have unprotected sex if she doesn't want a baby?
- Are pro-choice advocates saying that an embryo or fetus is not alive and human? How do they justify destroying that life when everywhere else in our culture, destroying [killing] an innocent life is a crime? It's a crime (feticide) for someone else to maliciously cause the death of an unborn human.
- What happens to the aborted embryos and fetuses?
- How much and specifically who profits from the abortion industry?
- Is the fact that Black and Hispanic women abort at higher rates than white women a form of minority population control?

Where Should We Go from Here?

Since the legalization of Roe v. Wade in 1973, over sixty-three million abortions occurred. Could it be that too many mothers and fathers have done a poor job educating their daughters (and sons), while abortion advocates did an excellent job propagandizing the "need" for abortions for any reason? The two combined create a definite advantage to the abortion industry, who is the only one profiting from how young women are choosing to use their bodies.

Our society tends to look at any view considered conservative as backward, wrong, even discriminatory. Yet if commonsense prevailed, could we see the value in young people looking at sexual relationships more responsibly? Afterall would an abortion be necessary if a woman made the choice not to get pregnant by changing her behavior, using contraceptives correctly and consistently and by knowing her ovulation cycle? What if women planned their pregnancies with their partner when both were ready and wanting to become parents, giving their child both a mother and father who wants them? What child wouldn't want that?

The facts are clear. One must take a hard detour from reality and the facts of fetal development to conclude that an abortion is just getting rid of a little "pregnancy tissue." It is killing a human life that is highly active and busy developing to get to the stage of life outside of the womb. But it is most definitively a human life inside the womb. We've coddled ourselves into using the antiseptic term of abortion rather than feticide, but the results are exactly the same – the death of a human being in the womb.

Women still have their reproductive rights and choices. Women in the US have the right to get pregnant anytime and by anyone they want, whether they can afford the child or not and whether they are prepared to be a mother. It is a choice. Women who choose to have random sex with strangers, or in "friends with benefits" relationships or are in committed monogamous relationships can all choose to learn about the contraceptive(s) best for them to prevent unwanted pregnancies from their healthcare provider. Then only the abortion providers would suffer.

Forgiveness and Hope After Abortion

Without a doubt some women experience remorse, guilt or even shame after having an abortion. Women may suffer trauma if coerced to abort by their partner or family members. Others realize that a preborn baby's life ended at their request. What woman cannot look back at the sexual encounter where she got pregnant and see in hindsight that the sex wasn't worth the outcome of an unwanted pregnancy? Others may have no remorse or regret at all.

For women who suffer after having an abortion it is imperative they forgive themselves and move forward living a positive purposeful life. There is no point in self-punishment about something that is now in the past. The best outcome for making a mistake in life is to not make it repeatedly. Everyone messes up sometime. Everyone has regrets about something they did they shouldn't have done or about something they should have done but didn't do. No woman should allow anyone to make her feel bad about having had an abortion- what's done is done. There is healing in loving and forgiving oneself.

Faith and Abortion

While women of faith may grapple with the decision to abort, it can be especially distressing for them who know their religion especially Judaism, Christianity, or Islam forbids sexual dalliances outside of marriage. Those three intertwined religions all affirm one eternally existing deity who is the Creator and Sustainer of all things including us human beings. For example, in the Bible, the book Christians believe as God's word and their handbook for life, there are consequences in our body to fornication and adultery (i.e., sexually transmitted diseases to unwanted pregnancies) and that God intended we engage in sex within the context of marriage.

Most people, whether religious or non-religious, might agree that adultery, murder, and stealing are all wrong. It's not hard to enumerate the negative consequences of each. Yet culturally we think that having sex outside of marriage is acceptable and waiting until marriage or at least a mutually exclusive committed love relationship is just old fashioned. Yet there are negative consequences to having multiple partners and relationships that are not monogamous (STDs, unwanted pregnancies, out of wedlock births often in poverty, abortions, higher cancer risks). Many Christians lack knowledge of what their Bible [they claim to believe in] says about those babies in the womb or they choose to ignore it and do what agrees with their social mores rather than their faith.

Women of all different faiths have abortions, regardless of what their doctrine dictates. Christianity, the faith of Protestants and Catholics as well as Judaism and Islam says that sex outside of marriage, both fornication and adultery is using the body sinfully.

Every person of faith should question their true beliefs whether they honestly believe their God as the creator of all things including humans. Or do they treat their God and the dictates of their faith as a menu, picking what they like from Column A and something else from Column B – thereby relegating their God to an idea of what they agree with sometimes and choosing to follow the current cultural mores at other times. Every person can decide for themselves if this passage from the Holy Bible in Psalm 139:13-18 (NLT*) resonates within them:

*[13]You [meaning God] made all the delicate, inner parts of my body and knit me together in my mother's womb.
[14] Thank you for making me so wonderfully complex! Your workmanship is marvelous—how well I know it.*

15 You watched me as I was being formed in utter seclusion,
as I was woven together in the dark of the womb.
16 You saw me before I was born.
Every day of my life was recorded in your book.
Every moment was laid out
before a single day had passed
17 How precious are your thoughts about me,[a] O God.
They cannot be numbered!
18 I can't even count them;
they outnumber the grains of sand!
And when I wake up,
you are still with me!

Children are a gift from the Lord, they are a reward from Him. Psalm 127:3 (NLT*)

*New Living Translation

Each of us has a free will to do as we choose, believe as we wish, as we experience the consequences that follow the choices we make.

How Can You Reduce Abortions?

Most reasonable people might agree that the fewer abortions performed, the better for everyone except those who profit from abortions. Women will have avoided unwanted pregnancies, unborn babies will not die, and the anxiety, fear, and expense all avoided. Who would not agree it is better for a woman to not get pregnant in the first place if she does not want a child? Whether you are pro-life or pro-choice there are things you can do to help prevent on demand abortions. Choose your level of involvement but do something.

1. Teach your own children and those you have influence over about pregnancy prevention and make them familiar with fetal development.
2. Encourage a sensitivity to respect human life and the importance of sexual responsibility. They should know that it is incredibly easy and smart not to get pregnant if they are not ready to have a child.
   a. Advise sexually active teens to use condoms 100% of the time.
   b. Instruct girls about their ovulation, the dozen or more contraceptives they can choose from and their efficacy rates.

c. Ask the teens and young women in your life what they would do if they got pregnant – there should be an emergency plan (emergency contraceptives, adoption?) to avoid abortion.

d. Check with the public schools in your area for what they are doing to teach pregnancy prevention other than abstinence. Approach schools and colleges to do more to inform girls and young women to avoid abortions by knowing how to avoid unwanted pregnancy, along with sexually transmitted infections, and using contraceptives. Boys too!

3. Join an organization that supports your views but do not be afraid to introduce the idea of pregnancy prevention (ask, "What's wrong with it, why aren't we doing more?").

4. Use your social media presence to talk about pregnancy prevention and reducing the number of abortions.

5. Write to your elected officials to make sure your state focuses on pregnancy prevention and the incredibly easy ways to learn the many contraceptive choices.

Finally, the Questions for Women

If a teen or young woman is not mature enough to evaluate and answer these questions for herself, she may not be ready to have sex and be responsible for the possible consequences:

- Is it better to prevent an unwanted pregnancy rather than get pregnant and then have an abortion?
- Have I learned about my body's ovulation and when I have the highest chance of getting pregnant?
- Have I consulted a healthcare professional to learn the best method(s) of birth control for me?
- Am I responsible enough to use the birth control method I've chosen consistently and correctly?
- Have I decided on what kind of sex life I want? *(Random hookups, committed exclusive relationship, marriage, casual relationships with more than one partner, etc.)*, and do I know the possible consequences in my body and for my life with my choices?
- Am I mature enough to discuss with my sexual partner what we would do if a pregnancy occurred? (Hint: If you can't talk

about it before you do it, you may not be mature enough to do it).

- Do I understand how a baby develops in the womb week by week and if I became pregnant what I would do?
- If I decided to get an abortion, how would I pay for it and who would I tell?
  - o Knowing the development stage of the baby, how would I feel afterwards?
- If I were to have a baby and keep it, how would I afford and raise him or her, especially if the father were not involved?
- If I had a baby could/would I be strong enough to give it up for adoption?
- Am I aware of the consequences of having sex with more than one person especially within a short time frame (e.g. – STDs, pregnancy. and not knowing who is the father).
- How do I feel about abstaining from sex for a period of time? What would I do instead?

Understand how humans develop in the womb by simply doing an internet search on *weekly fetal development* and find legitimate scientifically and medically factual information, such as:

Mayo Clinic, The Cleveland Clinic, and WebMD and others all provide legitimate, scientifically accurate information on pregnancy and fetal development.

An internet search on how abortions are performed results in dozens of sites (and viewpoints), some factual and medical, others opinionated.

To learn more facts about pregnancy, resources for the many options available for both pregnancy prevention and the options for an unintended pregnancy check out the American Pregnancy Association at https://americanpregnancy.org/

What If...?

What if we saw or heard public service announcements on the radio, tv, social media, everywhere with the presidents of pro-choice and pro-life organizations coming together to unite and advocate for women, for example:

As President of Planned Parenthood and President of the National Right to Life Committee our views on abortion differ, but we both believe and agree that preventing unwanted pregnancies is best for young women. We encourage sexually active women to visit their healthcare provider and learn about the best birth control method for them, understand how ovulation and pregnancy occur. Know that if you have unprotected sex or experience birth control failure the morning after pill also known as Plan B emergency contraception is 95% effective if taken within 24 hours to prevent a pregnancy from occurring. It is legal in all 50 states and available at grocery stores and pharmacies without a prescription. You do not have to get pregnant if you do not want to. We don't agree on everything, but we do agree that it is much better to protect yourself from an unwanted pregnancy, rather than facing one.

What a great woman-affirming unifying day for women's reproductive health that would be!

Study and Discussion Guide

Anyone can use this study/discussion guide for greater clarity on how and why they came to believe what they believe regardless of whether they are pro-choice or pro-life. As well as what their decision means to them personally. Both sides preach their own position, yet an individual does not have to pledge allegiance to either side. Instead, they can study the facts and incorporate their personal beliefs, their morals, and ethical values to be comfortable in their own mind that they have not allowed other's narratives to determine their position on abortion. Use it to assist teens and young adults to contemplate how and why they come to their beliefs, who or what influences them and how to make decisions for themselves using what they know to be true and factual.

Parents: Use the questions and scenarios in this discussion guide as conversation starters. Parents can use it to learn more about their teens and what influences them, what they believe and why.

Teachers: Design assignments using the questions for group or individual tasks and incorporate using critical thinking to investigate and analyze the facts on both sides of the abortion argument, where they can rationally explain both sides. Encouraging students to be open-minded and seek to problem-solve with those they do not agree with will help them mature in other facets of life be it academic or personal.

For Teens and Young Women

1. After studying weekly fetal development and relating it to how you developed in your mother's womb, does it alter or solidify your views on abortion? Explain how and why.

_____

_____

_____

_____

_____

_____

2. It's nearly impossible to draw a conclusion without being influenced by something or someone. Think about and write down how you came to believe your views on abortion and what influences from social media, your social group, family, friends, your moral, ethical or religious views and respected authority figures played a part.

_____

_____

_____

_____

_____

_____

3. Has studying both how a pregnancy occurs and develops and what happens when a fetus is aborted changed your views about abortion? Explain.

_____

_____

_____

_____

_____

_____

4. What do you think is the reason so many girls and young women choose abortion instead of preventing an unwanted pregnancy in the first place?

_____

_____

_____

_____

_____

_____

5. What do you think should happen to help teens and young women choose to prevent an unwanted pregnancy with the proper use of contraceptives instead of getting pregnant only to abort?

_____

_____

_____

_____

_____

_____

6. Who profits most from abortion?

_____

_____

_____

_____

7. Why do you think the pro-choice advocates who do not profit from abortion do not promote pregnancy prevention methods just as much or more as they promote abortion rights?

_____

_____

_____

_____

_____

_____

8. What are your thoughts on this: If a female has consensual unprotected sexual intercourse isn't she really trying to get pregnant (even if she claims to not want to get pregnant)? Explain your reasoning.

_____

_____

_____

_____

_____

_____

_____

9. What are your thoughts on the over one
   million abortions done annually? What do you
   think could have been done to prevent most
   of those unwanted pregnancies?

_____

_____

_____

_____

_____

10. Do you see any complexities in determining if a fetus is alive and human, and if so, what are they?

_____

_____

_____

_____

_____

_____

11. When you were rapidly developing in your mother's womb (review the week-by-week fetal development), do you think *you* were alive and human then? If not, at what stage of her pregnancy did you become alive and human? Ask your mother or someone who has had a child these same questions. Did they differ from your answer, how?

_____

_____

_____

_____

12. If you are sexually active (females and males), what precautions have you taken to prevent an unwanted pregnancy?

_____

_____

_____

_____

_____

_____

13. Do you know what ovulation is and its relevance in how pregnancy occurs? If not, what can you do to learn more about your own ovulation (females) or how a woman can determine her ovulation cycle (males)?

_____

_____

_____

_____

_____

_____

14. Research the various forms of contraceptives and name three and their rates of effectiveness in preventing pregnancy.

_____

_____

_____

_____

_____

_____

15. What are the various emergency contraceptives if a female had unprotected sex, or her birth control failed? Research emergency contraceptives, how they work, their effectiveness, availability, and cost.

_____

_____

_____

_____

_____

_____

_____

16. Why do you feel pro-choice advocates often use the terms *pregnancy tissue* or *fetus* and pro-life advocates may use the term *pre-born* or *baby* when they are both referring to a human being developing in the womb? Why do you think these terms make a difference to each group and what are they trying to accomplish with them?

_____

_____

_____

_____

_____

17. If you had to switch places with someone whose views were opposite to your views on abortion, how would you present their side from their viewpoint?

_____

_____

_____

_____

_____

18. Eight states and Washington DC allow abortions throughout a pregnancy (no limit). Review the fetal development stages from weeks 16-40. After 11 weeks a surgical abortion is required. Research on how late term abortions is performed in relation to the fetus's development. What are your thoughts?

_____

_____

_____

_____

_____

19. Should anyone other than the pregnant female and the male who impregnated her be financially responsible for an abortion or for the expenses of having a baby? Why or why not?

_____

_____

_____

_____

_____

_____

20. What are your thoughts on the extreme views some hold on abortion – abortions should be allowed even up until the birth of a baby, or no abortions should be allowed even to save the life of the mother or in the case of rape or incest?

_____

_____

_____

_____

_____

_____

21. Since an abortion ends a pregnancy, causing
    the death of an unborn human being, explain
    your thoughts on whether anyone should
    consider the unborn body when using the
    phrases, "a woman's right to choose," and
    "my body my choice?"

_____

_____

_____

_____

_____

22. How do you reconcile the logic between the
    act of feticide, a crime, and the act of an on-
    demand abortion chosen by the mother as
    both events result in the death of an unborn
    baby? Is one wrong and the other right?
    Explain.

_____

_____

_____

_____

_____

_____

23. Why do you think our culture has accepted on demand abortion as a reproductive right, when unwanted pregnancies are easily avoidable?

_____

_____

_____

_____

_____

_____

24. Review the section *What Does a Commonsense Abortion Policy Look Like* and discuss what if anything you agree with and

what you disagree with and would do differently. Explain your reasons.

_____

_____

_____

_____

_____

_____

_____

25. Some religious beliefs are that having sex without being married is wrong, and that there are many unwanted consequences for doing it, while others believe it to be old fashioned and out-of-date. What do you believe, why and what are the pros and cons of each view?

_____

_____

_____

_____

_____

_____

_____

26. What is the scientific reason why the more sexual partners a person has, the more they increase their chances of contracting a sexually transmitted disease (STD) or infection, some incurable?

_____

_____

_____

_____

_____

_____

_____

27. How do you explain the fact that an uninfected male and uninfected female in a sexual relationship only with each other cannot contract a STD?

_____

_____

_____

_____

_____

_____

28. For females: When (if ever) do you feel you
    would be ready to become pregnant and have
    a baby? Consider – *what you want to
    accomplish in life before becoming a mother,
    if you want to raise a child as a single mother
    or be married to the father first.*

_____

_____

_____

_____

_____

29. For males: When do you feel you would be
    ready to be a father? Consider -*what you
    want to accomplish in life, would you want to
    be married to the mother or be a single dad,*

and how you would support your child
physically, financially, emotionally.

_____

_____

_____

_____

_____

_____

_____

Decisions, Decisions, Decisions

It is common for young people to think about sex more around early to late teens in one way or another. As humans we are all sexual beings as it is the only way for people to continue –sexual intercourse between males and females is the only natural way to create more people.

While young people under the age of eighteen often want to "play around," sexually, it is advisable that both young males and females consider their family's values, the laws in their state regarding having sex as well as the consequences of pregnancy and the emotional decisions that come with it. Teens should know in advance what their family would do if they became pregnant or impregnated someone.

As one father told his teen-age son (goes for girls too), *"If you can't feed, clothe, and shelter, yourself and any baby you make with your own earnings you cannot afford to have sex. Sex is not going anywhere, there will be plenty of opportunities when you can be fully responsible for the consequences."* Something to think about.

For young males, having sex with someone under eighteen could have results that affect their lives much more than getting a girl pregnant depending on the age of consent in their state. Even consensual sex could result in criminal charges, jail time and/or having to register as a sex offender. All because they did not know the law and did not choose self-control. Just like it is okay for a girl to say no, it is also okay for a boy to say no to an underage girl. The law does not care that she says she had consensual sex.

For females: having sexual intercourse can result in pregnancy leaving her with a heart wrenching decision – abort, give away her baby, or keep her baby and raise it. Any one of the choices can affect her for the rest of her life.

Take time to think about how you want to live your life.

Write down how you want to take control of your sex life. Consider:

- How many partners you would like and why?
- Do you want to be promiscuous, have multiple random partners, wait until marriage, never marry?
- What are the consequences of having unprotected sex and how will you deal with them?
- Do you want to be in an exclusive committed relationship before having sex? If so, what will you do if the person you like wants to have sex but does not want to be exclusive with you?
- Are you afraid to say "no" or "not yet" to sex if it means your partner may leave and go to someone who says "yes?"

- Do you feel you are mature enough to discuss sex with your partner *before* doing it – what form of birth control will you use, condom use (helps prevent pregnancy and diseases), getting tested for STDs, what you would do if you (female) got pregnant or (male) impregnated someone?
- Do you agree or disagree with the parent's statement about not being able to afford the consequences of sex? Imagine you are a parent, what would you want your child to consider regarding their sex life?
- What is your action plan for preventing an unwanted pregnancy and protecting your sexual health considering what you want to accomplish in your life:

_____

_____

_____

_____

_____

_____

_____

About the Author

The Commonsense Citizen, Karen Lewis, is a woman who was deeply affected by the outrage after the Supreme Court overturned the Roe v. Wade decision. She could not help but see areas both sides could agree on but were too entrenched in "their side" to do so. She sees the chasm between the opposing sides as detrimental to women of childbearing age who are most affected by the decision to abort. But she also sees that by coming together we all could significantly reduce the number of elective abortions through pregnancy prevention. Karen is a long-time transplant to the Atlanta, Georgia area. There are other controversial issues in our culture that she sees a commonsense approach to, a way of coming together for the common good rather than continuing the spiraling divisiveness in our country. Look for more Commonsense Guides in the future, available on Amazon.com.

www.ingramcontent.com/pod-product-compliance
Lightning Source LLC
Chambersburg PA
CBHW050544280326
41933CB00011B/1720